ANTI-AGEING TIPS
HOW TO LOOK TEN TIMES YOUNGER THAN YOUR AGE

VICTORIA E.

DEDICATION

This book is dedicated to the Almighty God and my
online readers

CONTENTS

Chapter 1

Introduction

Growing older is a given. We must all accept this fact until a genetic fountain of youth is discovered.

With the knowledge that, as we age and add more years to the cake, our health will begin to degrade,
Okay, so the last part might not be entirely accurate. Once you reach a certain age, most individuals stop trying.
You do, however, have some control over how you age, even if it is unavoidable that you will become older. You have control over how you want to feel, look, and be physically healthy. Yes, some of this is luck, but a lot of it also has to do with what you eat, how you live, and even how you think. No matter what life throws at you, whether you're a man or a woman, you'll discover the key to aging gracefully.

You'll realize that pains, aches, and damaged skin are not inescapable and that your body can and should last you the rest of your life. And you'll discover how to continue thriving even after you leave this planet.

Who Is This Book For?

Before we continue, I want to stress that everyone can benefit from this Book.

It's possible that you feel that it's "too late" for you in some sense if you're already approaching your golden years. You might think it's too late to reverse your arthritis and wrinkles now that they've appeared. However, for younger readers, it will ultimately depend on your level of foresight. How well you can predict the future and make plans for it, instead of doing what makes you happy right now. But I want you to imagine a day in the future before you decide whether this is something you should spend your time on. This day could come about in a few years or a few decades. But eventually, your old school or college friends will probably phone you and invite you to a reunion. Now you can show up at that occasion looking amazing, if you're single, you can choose from all the sexiest people.

Chapter 2

Why it's Never Too Late to be What You Always Wanted to Be

You might be expecting me to immediately give you some advice on how to protect your skin. But allow me to say this: that is merely the surface. You can be sure that we'll address it later in this book because it's vital (and a sign of better overall health).
But what matters most is how you feel and the results you achieve.
Because how you feel about yourself and about life can greatly influence how you turn out, how people perceive you, and what you are capable of. You'll appear younger if you feel younger and that will make all the difference if you are energetic and excited about life.

When we decide to merely get by from day to day and give up on our aspirations, many of us will begin to physically age. The only way to maintain your youth and allure is to have a purpose in life and a goal to work toward.
You must, therefore, never let go of your goals. And there is really no incentive to do so...

How Age Affects Our Goals and Expectations
When we were younger, a lot of us aspired to accomplish incredible things. Some of us aspired to be

astronauts, some to be rock stars, and still others to be business men or women. Maybe you've always wanted to run your own company when you were in your twenties, though, the fact that you'll have had more time to amass beneficial assets is another factor that includes material things like money—you'll have more money to work with—as well as intangible and tangible assets like a home, connections, a stronger resume, etc. Additionally, you will have extra time if you are retired or if your children have moved out.

There's no reason you can't do things even as you get older if you put all of it together with a smart understanding of how to utilize your age.

Examples of Amazing Things You Can Still Do

For instance, many people wish to become actresses but never get around to it while they are younger. But when you're older, you can submit an application. Starting a profitable business at the age of 55 has twice the chances of starting at the age of 20-34?

Never surrender.

Naturally, staying physically fit, avoiding chronic pain, and maintaining a sharp, youthful mind will all help you take advantage of your possibilities at any age. You'll look younger thanks to your mindset and accomplishments, and you'll feel and perform better if you do. Therefore, we'll examine several strategies for maintaining your youthful appearance in the following chapter.

Chapter 3

How to Look Younger Than You Are

The types of advice you will get can be roughly divided into two groups when it comes to looking younger. On the one hand, you have suggestions that will center on how you can stop looking older. As they say, prevention is better than cure, so if you concentrate on taking care of your skin and avoiding aging habits, you can maintain your youthful appearance for years to come.
But that is not the topic of this chapter. The advice that will make you look younger when it's "already too late" is covered in this chapter. This chapter, which we're starting with it's the quickest and easiest, is all about hiding your current appearance.

Skin care products with vitamins and minerals can also be very beneficial, and some even have antioxidants that can be applied topically. Before making a decision, make sure to read, reviews and understand the science.

Getting a tan is an excellent additional tactic. By making your skin darker, a tan will help you conceal lines and wrinkles by reducing the contrast between the dark "shadows" where your lines are, and the rest of your skin.

This is not the goal because, as we'll discover in a later chapter, sun exposure is one of the main causes of skin aging more rapidly.

Search for "self-tanning moisturizers" instead. These underutilized products will naturally give your skin color and this is when taking a makeup lesson could be a terrific option. Classes like "Color Me Beautiful" can teach you how to use cosmetics expertly and to communicate with your face.

Tips for Achieving the Cougar/Milf Look.

You should now understand everything I have said, and you should be able to see how it might affect your capacity to appear and feel younger.

You may have also observed that there are some instances of women who deviate from this advice and nonetheless look fantastic. For instance, Teri Hatcher and the Desperate Housewives cast as a whole, Joanna Lumley, Courtney Cox, and Julie Bowen... These are young women who wear significantly darker makeup to appear younger than they are.

And shorter hair is an excellent approach to hiding forehead flaws for both men and women. Help cover gray hairs or replace hair that you might be losing. Try shaving the sides and growing your hair out longer on top.

Men who are balding should not oppose the process. A

weak comb over is among the most unpleasant things, and you are nearly always better off adopting a shaved head. If anything, it will make you appear more rugged. Here's an example of how you can "work" your appearance as an older man. While softness, suppleness, and youthfulness are the hallmarks of classic female beauty, men can get away with seeming tough but this is frequently overlooked, so keep your hands moisturized to avoid that oversight!

Dress Age-Proof.

The goal is not to dress youthfully in order to appear youthful, just like with makeup and hair color. You should dress for your age if you wish to appear younger. Work your look; don't try to change it.

Hydrate

Hydration is one of the single most crucial steps you can take to look younger right away. Dehydration can make our skin appear thinner because it causes less water to be retained under the surface. This makes veins under the skin easier to detect, and it also makes wrinkles more obvious.

Many of us appear dehydrated because we are dehydrated.

A simple way to take years off of you is to get them taken care of. That could entail seeing the hygienist to have them cleaned or requesting that they be made whiter. Also keep in mind that missing teeth can cause your mouth to become more wrinkled.

As a result, while it may be uncomfortable, getting

permanent dentures (dental implants) to replace missing teeth is one of the best ways to appear younger.

Chapter 4

How to Look Younger for Longer

Chapter 4 provided nearly complete instructions on how to instantly appear younger. You should be if you followed that advice as you went, you might now have a haircut, clothes, and personal style that are more suitable. You might have discovered methods to make your skin look younger and to lessen the visibility of wrinkles and creases.

The time has come to advance further, though, It's time to stop the unrelenting passage of time from eroding your appearance even further. As we previously stated, prevention is preferable to treatment. How can you stop yourself from looking older, then?

The Best Aging Prevention Technique: Antioxidants. Foods that contain antioxidants operate by scavenging free radicals. In the meantime, free radicals are molecules that drinking acidic tap water regularly can result in significant oxidative damage over time. Installing a water ionizer will make all of your water less likely to cause oxidative damage, which will help you prevent wrinkles and significantly boost your energy levels.

According to studies, this has the potential to increase

lifespan and reduce outward signs of aging. Many people say that they begin to feel the effects within 30 days.

Glutathione, The Master Antioxidant

Do you need another expert anti-aging tip?

Try including a little bit more glutathione in your diet. This is the so-called "master antioxidant," as it is frequently referred to. It is a tripe tide comprised of cysteine, glutamine acid, and glycine.

Finally, be aware of how stress affects your cells, your brain, and your aging in a very bad way. Chronic stress opens the door for degradation, sickness, and accelerated aging. You encourage further inflammation. Your immune system, along with digestion and nutrient absorption, are all suppressed by stress, which also raises your heart rate. It enhances oxidative damage and induces inflammation. Therefore, if you can't escape it, learn how to deal with it. For all these reasons, meditation is one of the most effective techniques for delaying aging.

Skincare and nutrition

Last but not least, make sure you are taking good care of your skin as you age with the correct products and foods.

Chapter 5

Staying Fit and Healthy As You Age

Since the creation of the movie "Rocky," Stallone has been one of my personal heroes.
He also wrote the script himself.

Despite having no prior acting experience, he was able to perform the major role, get into great shape, and inspire bodybuilders and boxers all over the world.
Sly keeps wowing us today. At the ripe old age of 66, he may be in the best physical shape of his life and shows no signs of slowing down. He's old enough to be a granddad, but he still resembles his physique from the 1980s, which is very motivating for anyone approaching their senior years.
Not that you have to follow in their footsteps, but these supplements, which include things like Tribulus terrestris and Tongkat ali, have no known advantages for younger men. Despite the fact that testosterone production declines with age,

You'll discover that a supplement can help you tremendously if your health starts to suffer. Of course,

this is only applicable to men.
A lot of elderly men and women could benefit from producing more growth hormone, which will have similar effects. Although there isn't a simple way to add growth hormone, you can still promote production by working your legs with squats and going on rapid runs. Similarly, getting more rest and taking hot baths can help increase output. It's a hard pill to swallow, but it's for your health!
But joints are suffering a great deal. Finding low-impact exercises like swimming, walking, or riding a recumbent bike is the apparent solution.
Energy

Even with your body operating at full capacity, exercising as you age is challenging because you'll probably feel much more exhausted and out of energy when you come to do it. However, if you discover that you are experiencing this, you can always boost your energy by taking better supplements or by just getting more sleep and rest.
Go easy on your next workout if your muscles are still sore from your last one, and make sure you receive plenty of rest and protein before you focus on the same area once more.
and allow

Chapter 6

Your Brain – Keeping Your Mind Sharp as You Age

Growing older has a lot of unpleasant side effects, and there are a lot of reasons not to welcome the unavoidable march of time. While many of the negative aspects of aging that we prefer to focus on have to do with our bodies failing us, it may be even worse when our minds begin to falter and we notice that we are forgetful and think much more slowly.
Even if we don't necessarily have a specific illness like dementia, we may still notice that we are thinking more slowly and finding it difficult to keep up with everyone else, which may be quite unpleasant and isolating. However, if you are prepared to put in the time and effort, it doesn't have to be that way.

Memory. This kind of memory, which is frequently lost as you get older, is essential for having "fluid intellect."

Diet

The appropriate diet can work wonders for protecting your brain health and assisting in delaying the beginning of some neurological illnesses or general decline. Fatty acids like omega 3 that you can receive through seafood and supplements are very helpful.

Omega-3 fatty acids can reduce inflammation, which can harm the brain, as well as boost "cell membrane permeability," which improves communication between neurons. Amino acids (proteins), which you can acquire through meat or supplements, and vitamins like B9 (also known as folic acid), which are found in fruits and vegetables, are used to stress and sleep deprivation both exacerbate physical and mental damage, speed up cell death, and deteriorate your immune system.

Immunological response.

Finally, take into account something that is frequently disregarded: brain injury. Traumatic brain injury and the beginning of conditions like Parkinson's and dementia are strongly correlated.

Boxers and other athletes frequently sustain brain injuries that have a severe impact on their health as they get older. Similarly, many of us may sustain injuries from slips, trips, and other events that will result in subtle alterations to our brains that we will not realize. Many of us are currently coping with mild brain injuries. Wear helmets, stay away from jolting contact sports, and so keep expanding your knowledge. Continue to push yourself to pick up new abilities, talents, and programming languages, and continue making new friends. Continue exploring new locales. And

Persistently pursue your goals. Always keep in mind that it is never too late to pursue your dreams.

Chapter 7

The Future: Has the First Person to Live Forever Already Been Born?

Did you know that a species of jellyfish exists that is biologically immortal? It could theoretically live indefinitely and never die unless physically killed by a predator or disease.

This is conceivable due to the jellyfish's ability to "revert" back into its "polyp" shape, much like Dr. Who, and regenerate all of its cells in the process. This jellyfish is known as Turritopsis nutricula. Personally, I think that this is the most likely means by which people will pass away, but it is irrelevant right now.

The argument is that, despite the possibility that humanity will someday achieve biological immortality, most scientists think that the first person to live forever has most likely already been born. How is that even possible? How, for instance, a recent study by the Institute of Regenerative Medicine in Pittsburgh showed that injecting mice with stem cells from younger mice could extend their lives by 200%. This has already been proven successful.

It's likely only a matter of time until comparable procedures are tested on humans after working efficiently on mice. Certainly not 140 years...
Other strategies for extending human life have also been put forth. For example, the durability and functionality of mitochondria—the energy-producing "batteries" that surround our cells and shield them from oxidative damage—have been improved using gene doping techniques.
According to predictions, these medicines could lengthen our lives by up to 30% while also enhancing our protection.